Holistic
EMOTIONAL
INTELLIGENCE

Holistic
EMOTIONAL
INTELLIGENCE

SET YOUR MIND,
IT'S ALL ABOUT ENERGY!

DR. WANDA BONET-GASCOT

To order additional copies of this book, please contact:
Palibrio
1663 Liberty Drive
Suite 200
Bloomington, IN 47403
Toll Free from the U.S.A 877.407.5847
Toll Free from Mexico 01.800.288.2243
Toll Free from Spain 900.866.949
From other International locations +1.812.671.9757
Fax: 01.812.355.1576
orders@palibrio.com
794099

CONTENTS

Dedication vii

Gratitude.. ix

Preface xi

Foreword.. xv

Introduction: The Backstage Story xix

Part I: Energy Consciousness................................... 1

Part II: Energy Vitality... 7

Part III: Energy Harmony 36

Part IV: Energy Alignment..................................... 73

Part V: Energy Communion *"Mobius"*................... 79

Conclusion 83

Bonus: Holistic Emotional Intelligence
Coaching Method © 85

About the Author 93

References & Resources... 95

Dedication

Dedicated to you, Reader!

"The heart of the prudent acquires knowledge,
and the ear of the wise seeks knowledge"
Proverbs 18:15

Gratitude

Thank God for wisdom, understanding, communication, strength, knowledge, compassion and courage to handle my emotions in a healthy way and carry this message to humanity.

Thanks to my children, Carlos Juan & David; and my life partner, Carlos Chinea.

Thanks to my mentors, colleagues, students, and clients.

Thanks to you, reader, for existing...

FOREVER THANK YOU!

> *"I am what I am, and that's all that I am" – Popeye*

Preface

It would be wonderful if we could plan our lives from the beginning so everything would turn just as we anticipated. We would be able to reach our goals without tripping on the way while being in full control of our environment, achieving the golden future we all wish for, aspire to and deserve to have.

Life, however, is quite different. We can plan for diverse goals and work very hard to attain them, but that is no guarantee that we will reach our original plans unscathed. As we walk through this trail we will find both ample avenues and dead ends; wonderful detours that could shorten our journey or make us arrive to it unprepared. Let's remember that in order to enjoy the sweet flavor of a fruit we should not take it from the tree before it is ready. We will encounter road junctions, each path as promising as the next one...but we will also find cliffs with no return in which we need to walk very carefully because one false step can make a difference between keeping on walking or falling down the ravine. It is during those moments when we make changes in our navigation plan to readjust our route and arrive to secure port.

We seem to believe that this "port" we aspire to arrive to is where the final goal lies. We come to this world with an emotional devise which tells us that our paths must be directed towards this so much valued and idealized happiness that we obtain through self-realization. And while there is some truth in this, there might be some points of adjustment. Happiness is not found in a specific place… for several reasons. Because it is relative to our beliefs, desires and goals; because we forget that in any equation there are variables beyond our control that could alter the expected results. Results are the product of our actions but we do not always succeed the first time, nor the second nor the third; sometimes we just can't come up with the solution. From this perspective we could infer that only a few will arrive to this "Safe Harbor". A bit pessimistic thought if we believe that being happy is our right.

Wouldn't it be better to make adjustments to our original emotional devise? To believe that we should be happy while we are in the road instead of walking to find happiness? To internalize that happiness is a state of the soul and not a goal in a senseless Olympiad? Because life is not a competition...life is a treasure!

This is not a manifest to teach you how to live your life. More than anything it is about tools, so that you may be able to walk towards the future with full conscience of your possibilities and with control of your steps, your own personal rhythm and your Safe Harbor, your Peace.

Edwin Ocasio
Entrepreneur of the Year 2017
Society of Emotional Intelligence
Orlando, FL

Foreword

I remember two things about the first time I met Dr. Wanda. First, her energetic and welcoming smile and second, her invitation to attend her monthly night meetings. Little did I know that, with my attendance, she would change my life. I took every training class she offered in her ***DRW Life Skills Institute & Coaching School,*** but more valuable to me, is the amazing friendship we share.

When Wanda says, "It's all about energy," she not only means it, she personifies. She lives energy. She exudes energy, but most importantly, she energizes her environment and the people in it. She is easily the most fascinating person I know, and by the simple act of reading this book, you too, will know this amazing woman.

In this very special, easy to read, short and to the point book, Wanda satiates the reader with the keys to unlocking his/her seldom tapped storehouse of energy. In just a few more than 100 pages, Wanda, shows you where your energy hides, how to find it, and best of all, how to use it to benefit not only yourself, but everyone you interact with.

Building on the well-established foundation of Emotional Intelligence, Wanda leads you on a unique and exciting journey into energized, personal excellence.

Finding your energy begins with Self-awareness. Hard as it is to believe, very few people really take the time to get acquainted with their real selves. In this chapter, Wanda helps you ask and answer several critical questions leading to a unique discovery of who you really are and where your undiscovered treasure troves of energy are hidden. Her theme in this chapter is, *"Energy Consciousness."* By the time you've finished the chapter, Wanda leads you to an excited awareness of how much better you can be. Are you getting excited? Well, you should be!

With the boundaries of self-awareness firmly built, Dr. Wanda moves on, in the next chapter, towards self-management or, as she says, *Energy Vitality.* Here she shows you how to increase the energy you have discovered by integrating new habits into your lifestyle. The energy is infinite; therefore, you have all your life to increase it and enjoy it.

Now that you know how to increase your energy, you are ready to immerse yourself in the *Energetic Harmony.*

You will be able to identify the ways in which the habits formed, the beliefs fed and the doubts about yourself have blocked your energy and, consequently, have limited your progress in life. This chapter demands honesty. This chapter requires identifying what you need to do less, but also more. This chapter shows you how to recognize and overcome the walls of the imagined negative reality that you have built around you. This chapter prepares you for the lessons in the next chapter on how to get along better with people. Most of us sail through life with little if any awareness of what is going on in the lives of those around us. We are often so self-absorbed that we ignore signs of sadness and often miss signals of happiness we would otherwise be invited to share. Dr. Wanda puts her decades of study in the field of Emotional Intelligence to work for you. The roadmap to better relationships is open to you. Read it. Learn from it, and follow it right in to the next chapter where she shows you how to build the kinds of relationships that energize you and the people you interact with.

Our ability to succeed in life is primarily tied to how well we get along with people. This chapter, entitled, Interpersonal Relationships, *Energy Alignment,* teaches you to apply what you've learned so far. In it, Dr. Wanda tells you to measure and value your relationships based on the level of energy you share, but also receive. She shows you how to align yourself with people whose energy compliments yours. In no uncertain terms she will tell you two essential things about mutually satisfying relationships. First, be a source of energy to everyone you spend time and second, avoid spending much time with people who drain you of energy. Wanda will tell you how to measure the energy level of each person you meet. She offers techniques for bringing their energy into alignment with yours. She shows you how energy alignment leads to great accomplishments.

Finally, in the chapter titled, *Energy Communion,* Dr. Wanda shares options to raise your energy frequency and strengthen your natural magnetism.

I asked you earlier if you are excited yet. I told you that you should be. I echo that in closing. There is much to be excited about hidden the pages of this little book. But even though the nuggets of wisdom are hidden, they are incredibly easy to find. Read the book, find your energy and learn to control and apply it. You'll be glad you did. Learning from Dr. Wanda has made my life and relationships so much better. Let her do that for you. Again, read this book.

-**Coach Dale Lind**
Emotional Intelligence Ambassador 2015
Society of Emotional Intelligence
Orlando, FL

Introduction:
The Backstage Story

What do you want? What's your goal?

Improve your health? Increase your productivity? Enjoy mutually satisfying interpersonal relationships?

Set your mind…It's all about energy!

Twenty years ago, I learned about the concept of Emotional Intelligence (EQ) while working as a chemist in a pharmaceutical industry in Puerto Rico. I fell in love with the four EQ pillars (self-knowledge, self-management, social awareness and interpersonal relations). I decided to integrate them into my personal and professional life.

Later, in 2004, I discovered and consciously felt energy for first time. It was an eye-opening experience, and my scientific mindset motivated me to learn more about it. The concept of energy fascinated me, and I decided to study Chinese Medicine, Energy Medicine and Energy

Modalities. In 2011, I completed a doctoral degree in Holistic Nutrition and Energy Medicine.

After several years of clinical practice, it all made sense. I remembered Albert Einstein, and his radical formula $E = mc^2$. For Einstein, energy and matter were the same only manifested in different forms. *"Everything is energy"*, he said, and he was right.

Emotions are energy in movement, and if they are not managed properly it causes stagnation, and energy stagnation causes illness and psychosomatic conditions. If we manage emotions properly, we will enjoy better health, more productivity, and mutually satisfactory interpersonal relationships.

In 2012, I coined the _Holistic Emotional Intelligence_ concept and published my first book: _Why am I not happy,_ as an introduction to the topic.

The feedback received sharing the _Holistic Emotional Intelligence_ concept motivated me to establish: *DRW Life Skills Institute & Coaching School*. In 2013, the institute was officially opened to share the **Holistic Emotional Intelligence Coaching Method**© in a structured and uniform way under the University of Central Florida, Business Incubator Program's umbrella.

Finally, after 15 years of researching, studying, experiencing and practicing energy, the book is ready: _Holistic Emotional Intelligence: Set your mind… It's all about Energy!_ This book presents the results of my research about energy, and its objective is to create awareness about energy consciousness, vitality, harmony, alignment, and communion. You will find techniques for developing emotional mastery, powerful approaches to feel your energy, effective ways to increase your energy and practical forms to unblock your energy centers, therefore, harmony, alignment, and experience **_"Mobius"_**.

Holistic Emotional Intelligence is the ability to use emotional information in an effective and conscious way to identify areas of improvement; to handle emotional triggers properly, to reduce energy stagnation and therefore enjoying better health, more productivity and mutually satisfactory interpersonal relationships.

Energy Consciousness Discover and Feel your Energy	***Energy Vitality*** Increase and Recharge your Energy
Energetic Harmony Unblock and Protect your Energy	***Energy Alignment*** Expand and Enjoy your Energy
Energy Communion Vibrate Higher and Experience Mobius	

The ***Emotional Holistic Intelligence*** model recognizes that emotions are energy in motion and that mismanaged emotions cause energy stagnation and energetic wear, both of which negatively impact our health, productivity and interpersonal relationships.

Enjoy your energy journey and remember,
What do you want? What's your goal?
Set your mind… *"It's all about energy"* –Dr. W

Part I

Energy Consciousness

Discover and Feel your Energy

Objective:

The aim of this chapter is to facilitate *Energy Consciousness* offering practical approaches to discover and feel your own energy.

Discover and Feel your Energy:

Energy is a concept that is used in the ordinary sense to designate the vigor or activity of a person, object or organization. Also, energy is the essential vital force that animates all life forms of the universe.

Whether the concept of energy is new to you or you are familiar with it; it is important to define energy in terms of *Holistic Emotional Intelligence*. ***Energy is the fuel for better health, more productivity, and mutually satisfactory interpersonal relationships.***

In order to start this journey, you must discover and feel your energy. "*Qigong*", a medicinal therapy of Chinese origin based on respiration, as a source of energy; offers an effective technique to feel the energy.

Steps to feel the energy:

1. Stand up with your feet apart from the distance of your shoulders.

2. Rub your hands quickly for about a minute.

3. Breathe deeply.

4. Keep your hands in front of you, with your palms facing inward, until they are separated at about 30cm. When you inhale, you put your hands

together more, but without touching them, and when you breathe out, turn them away again.

5. When the energy begins to accumulate in your hands, you will begin to feel a feeling of warmth and tingling.

6. Feel the magnetic force or heat in your hands until you feel a "ball" of accumulated energy in your hands, then play with the energy until you develop a relationship with it.

Congratulations, you've just discovered and felt your energy. It may seem extraordinary to feel the energy in your hands, imagine being able to feel or be aware of the energy around your body. In basic terms, the energy around your body is known as the aura, or electromagnetic field. It is luminous energy that surrounds all living beings in an oval form and is imperceptible in full view and extends between one and three feet away from the physical body in all directions. It's fascinating to feel it.

Another option to feel energy is to experience energy modalities. In my private practice, we offer *energy massages* and *singing bowls vibration therapy,* both are powerful opportunities to experience your bodies true energy.

One more way to discover your energy is imagining that you are the battery of your cell phone. Then, respond to the following questions:

1. What is your energy level? Zero (0) to one hundred (100). What is your energy percentage right now? 25%? 50%? 60%? 75%? 100%?

2. When was the last time you felt 100%? Where was it? What were you doing?

3. Close your eyes and feel the energy running through your body. Give yourself a chance to feel. Establish this moment as your baseline.

After having discovered and felt your energy, would you be interested in increasing it? If the answer is yes, I invite you to continue the learning and explore options to develop **Energy Vitality.**

Exercise:

1. From 0% 100%, where do you find yourself energetically at this moment?

2. What does your answer mean? Define

3. From 0% 100%, what energy level do you want to achieve?

4. What does your answer mean? Define

5. From 0 to 10, where 10 is fully committed and 0 means not being compromised; How committed are you to increase your energy levels?

Part II

Energy Vitality

Increase and Recharge your Energy

Objective:

The objective of this chapter is to facilitate *Energy Vitality* offering fifteen (15) effective options to increase and recharge your energy.

Increase and Recharge Your Energy

Strengthening your energy must be an intentional and daily process. Based on my years of study and research, the following fifteen (15) options are very effective to increase and recharge your energy.

1. Deep and Long Breathing
2. Effective Hydration
3. Conscious Diet
4. Physical Activity
5. Intentional Rest
6. Meditation or Prayer
7. Healthy Sexual Activity
8. Hobbies
9. Love
10. Read
11. Listen
12. Associate
13. Generate Passive Income
14. Living your Life Purpose
15. Living a Holistic Lifestyle

Effective Options to Increase and Recharge your Energy

1. _Long and Deep Breathing_

Did you know that the most cost-efficient way of our body to produce energy is by breathing?

Respiration is the main source of oxygen for our optimal performance. Therefore, the longer and deeper our breath is, the more oxygen we are supplying our cells to produce energy.

The air is made up of various gases, where only 21% is oxygen. The amount of energy that produces our body is proportional to the amount of oxygen we receive.

To increase your levels of energy breathes consciously in places of low environmental pollution.

2. _Effective Hydration_

Did you know that drinking ionized water is the most effective way to increase your energy?

Water is the main component of our body and represents near 70% of the body weight. The water is composed of two hydrogen molecules and one oxygen molecule. Oxygen is the main ingredient in energy production.

Every cell and every system in your body depends on water: either to transport nutrients, to remove toxins or to keep certain organs and tissues hydrated.

Although there are many recommendations for water we should drink, there is no set amount for all people. Remember we are unique, and our water intake is unique. Learn to listen to your body, if you are thirsty, that is a message that your body is dehydrated, meaning, you need water to be able to fulfill all vital functions.

Instead, when we talk about water quality, there are three (3) chemical properties that determine the efficiency of water in your body. Not all waters are equal in terms of effectiveness for energy production. Based on my personal and professional experience, the most effective water for energy production is *alkaline, ionized and high in antioxidants.*

Alkaline:

Acidity or alkalinity is measured by a universal scale graduated from 0 to 14 is 7 the neutrality point. Drinking alkaline water daily helps to maintain our alkaline internal environment, which encourages energy production. In alkalinity condition the body works better, the immune system works better, therefore we are healthier. On the other hand, acidity gives rise to diseases. It has been shown that diseases, including cancer, cannot live in an alkaline medium whereas, on the contrary, they develop in acidic environments.

Ionized

Water is a polar molecular, so it is agglomerated in groups of 10 to 13 molecules affecting the absorption process of our body. The membranes allow the entry of molecules according to their size. Ionized water has sizes of groups of smaller molecules facilitating the process absorption, therefore the hydration of our body and the production of energy.

Antioxidant Power

Antioxidants protect the body from the action of free radicals, which are especially reactive molecules capable of damaging the body through a process called oxidation. The most effective way to combat the negative effect of free radicals is to drink water with high anti-oxidant power.

To increase your energy levels, drink ionized water, alkaline and high in anti-oxidants, my choice is Kangen water.

For information about Kangen Water visit, <u>www. DRWinstitute.org</u>

3. *Conscious Diet:*

Did you know that our body uses energy to digest everything we consume?

Food is extremely important in the production of energy. To eat with energetic consciousness, you must know the properties of what you ingest.

The western way of eating is too heavy; food and beverages that consume a lot of energy during digestion.

Energetically conscious people:

I)   Eat lightly and energy-rich, including pure foods, which include all kinds of fruits, cereals, legumes, vegetables, and dairy. Do not consume artificial foods that contain colorants or preservatives. The body uses too much energy to clean itself and detox.

II)   Avoid refined foods such as white flour, rice, and sugar; instead they will consume integrals. The body expends energy by digesting those foods and does not receive any nutritional value in return.

III) Eat foods that are in their season and place of harvest to receive more nutritional value from the food.

IV) Chew thoroughly at least 40 times so they can be easily digested. The smaller the pieces of food easier to digest and absorb, therefore, the less energy will be used when digesting.

V) They eat only when they are hungry, to saturate the organism with foods that they cannot assimilate. Every time you ingest a food the body invests energy in the process of digestion, less food intake means we are more efficient with our energy. They don't eat before they go to sleep. The lighter we go to sleep, the more energy the body has for its restoration and internal healing.

VI) Eat in a serene and pleasant atmosphere. Eating in a healthy and calm environment offers good vibes to our body and saves us the energy of having to protect ourselves from the constant bombardment of negative frequencies.

VII) They eat breakfast like a king, lunch like a prince, and dine like a beggar. This principle is consistent with the biological clock recommended in traditional Chinese medicine. At night it is better to eat little to not overburden the digestive system and that the organism can devote itself to other functions.

VIII) They eat meditatively and devote all your attention and energy to the pleasurable act of eating.

Fasting

Fasting is the willing abstinence or reduction from some or all food, drink, or both, for a period. An **absolute fast** or **dry fasting** is normally defined as abstinence from all food and liquid for a defined period. Water fasting refers to abstinence from all food and drink except water, but black coffee and tea may be consumed. Other fasts may be partially restrictive, limiting only particular foods or substances, or be intermittent.

To increase your energy levels, consciously eat foods with high nutritional value and fast periodically.

4. *Physical Activity*

Did you know that physical activity influences your energy levels?

Performing physical activity increases circulation of oxygen in our body and therefore the production of energy. In general, physical activity or exercises is classified into four main categories: resistance, strength, balance, and flexibility.

Resistance

Endurance exercises increase the health of the heart, lungs and circulatory system. The physical activities that develop the resistance include walking fast, working in the garden, dancing, jogging, swimming, cycling, climbing stairs or climbing hills, among others.

Strengthening

Strengthening exercises increase muscle strength. Strengthening exercises include lifting weights and using a resistance band, among others.

Balance

Balancing exercises help prevent falls. Exercises to improve balance include standing on one foot and Tai Chi, among others.

Tai Chi is a martial art that offers benefits, both on a corporal and a mental level. All the muscles of the body are worked on, and other factors such as strength, flexibility, and balance are considered.

Flexibility

Stretching exercises can help your body stay flexible and agile. To increase flexibility, try the following exercises stretching the shoulders and upper arms, stretching the calves and yoga, among others.

Yoga originates in India more than 5000 years ago, yoga flexibility exercises are smooth and are movements that help to improve the length of the muscles, increasing the range of movement in the joints.

To increase your energy levels, do physical activity that stimulates circulation in your body.

5. *Intentional Rest*

Did you know your body recharges energetically while you rest?

Resting is vital to recharge energy and produce energy. There are many ways to rest intentionally. Evaluate the options and consciously integrate resting in your lifestyle.

Power Naps

Need to recharge? Don't lean on caffeine -- a power nap will boost your memory, cognitive skills, creativity, and energy level.

Recommendations for an effective power nap:

1. Find a good place to take a nap, where nobody interrupts you.
2. Choose a dark room or wear a sleeping mask.
3. Make sure it is not too hot or cold in the place.
4. Choose the duration of the nap.
5. Sleeping for twenty minutes is what most people consider a "power nap" and is ideal for most people.
6. Turn off your cell phone and other possible distractions.
7. Place a "do not disturb" sign outside your door or communicate your "nap" culture.
8. Set an alarm to rescue you, it will help you to relax as you will know that you will not sleep more than you want.
9. Close your eyes and relax.
10. Enjoy your power nap.

Energy Modalities

Energy modalities are a very effective way to increase your energy and recharge yourself. There are several modalities, among them; energy massages, Tibetan singing bowls and reiki. It is important to explore options and evaluate which option is best for you.

Biomat Therapy

One way to rest intentionally is using the **amethyst BioMat** for just a short time each day. It leaves your body relaxed and refreshed, and it's designed to fit your lifestyle. Whether you choose short or more prolonged periods, use it before bed-time to prepare your body for sleep, or incorporate the **BioMat** into your fitness, relaxation, health or meditation routine.

The core of the **BioMat** technology is a combination of far infrared rays, negative ion and the conductive properties of amethyst channels. These three powerful health stimulators are combined in a single, easy-to-use product with remarkable benefits. It's a safe and natural way to recharge your energy.

For information about Biomat technology, visit www. DRWinstitute.org

Sleep

Sleep is vital for good health. During sleep, physiological processes such as secretion of hormones in the metabolism, and cardiovascular, respiratory and immunological functions vital to our body occur.

Understanding the sleep cycle allows us to maximize the benefits of rest and to enjoy greater levels of energy.

The night Sleep is organized in 4 or 5 cycles comprised over approximately 8 hours. Each cycle lasts from 90 to 120 minutes and comprises 5 different stages: 1, 2, 3, 4, and REM sleep (rapid eye movement). These stages progress cyclically from 1 to REM then begin again with Stage 1.

Early sleep cycles each night have relatively short rem dreams and long periods of deep sleep but later in the night, REM periods lengthen, and deep sleep time shortens.

Stage 1 is the lightest part of the sleep and can be easily awakened. During this stage, many people experience sudden muscle contractions preceded by a feeling of falling.

Stage 2, eye movement stops, and brain waves become slower with only an occasional burst of fast brain waves.

In Stage 3, there are extremely slow brainwaves called Delta waves that are interspersed with smaller, faster waves.

In Stage 4, the brain produces delta waves almost exclusively. Stages 3 and 4 are referred to as deep sleep, and it is very difficult to awaken someone from them. When we find ourselves in deep sleep, there is no eye movement or muscle activity.

The REM (Rapid Eye Movement) stage is when the breathing becomes faster, superficial and irregular, the eyes are rapidly agitated, and the muscles of the limbs are temporarily paralyzed. Brainwaves during this stage are like those experienced by people being awake, heart rate increases, blood pressure rises, men experience erections, and the body loses some of the ability to regulate its temperature. It is the time that most dreams occur, if a person is awakened during REM sleep, he may be able to remember dreams. Most individuals experience three to five intervals of REM sleep each night.

Getaways

How often do you give yourself a break – a proper chance to recuperate and recharge your batteries? Busy schedules demand so much attention that some people never stop, but this can be detrimental to our physical and mental health, productivity and even relationships. A getaway is a short duration vacation designed to recharge your energy.

Benefits of a weekend getaway:

1. A chance to unwind: Getting away from the house puts a stop to constant reminders of the chores that need to be done and escaping from the office every now and again protects workers from burnout,

helping them to be more creative and productive on their return.

2. Health Benefits: Stress is not all in the mind – it can also have devastating effects on the body if you do not give yourself time to relax.

3. Spend quality time with quality people: A short break will give you plenty of time to spend with the people that you don't get to see enough, whether that is a partner, family or friends.

4. Practical considerations: In the current economic climate, weekend breaks are more finance friendly and are less likely to cause you money-related stress on your return.

For information about our *3 Day / 2 Night All Inclusive Energy Weekend Retreat,* visit www.DRWinstitute.org

Vacations

Vacation is an extended period of leisure and recreation, especially one spent away from home or in traveling. Taking vacations is essential, not only for our wellbeing, but for maintaining sanity while back at home.

Benefits of vacations

1. **Stress reduction:** Vacations work to reduce stress by removing people from the activities and environments that they associate with stress and anxiety.

2. **Improved productivity.** Vacations make you happy. When you're happier, you excel at what you do.

3. **Better sleep.** Vacations can help interrupt the habits that disrupt sleep, like working late into the night or watching a backlit screen before bed. If you have stress from work and you find your sleep is disrupted because of anxiety or tension, take time off and learn to reset your sleep pattern. Take some time off so you can sleep better and be more productive, more relaxed, and healthier. It is a very recharging intentional rest.

To increase your energy levels, take time off and rest intentionally.

6. _Meditation and/or Prayer_

Did you know meditation and/or prayer stimulates the immune system and the mechanisms of healing?

The term meditation and/or prayer refers to a broad spectrum of practices that include techniques designed to promote relaxation, build internal energy or life force. The meditation and/or prayer takes different meanings in different contexts; this has been practiced since antiquity as a component of many religions and beliefs. The basic foundations of effective prayer are an act of grace, adoration, confession, petition, and intersection.

For many people, it's a little bit hard the meditation process, but intentional and conscious practice helps to develop the habit and enjoy its benefits.

Here are some basic recommendations to start meditating:

- Choose a quiet environment
- Put on comfortable clothes
- Follow your breath
- Repeat a mantra
- Try to meditate at the same time every day

To increase your energy levels integrates meditation and/or prayer into your lifestyle.

7. *Healthy Sexual Encounter*

Did you know that we can reach exponential levels of energy during a sexual encounter?

Sexual activity is one of the most effective ways to enjoy the energy. It is achieved by the activation of the second energy center and/or through energy alignment "Mobius". The sexual energy is creation energy, it is sacred. Two is always more than one. The amount of energy reached will be proportional to the amount of energy that each one brings to the encounter. It is important to recognize the intention during the sexual encounter. There are options for learning the art and science of sacred sexuality, it is your responsibility to evaluate the option or combination of options that resonate with your essence and your moral values. For example, Tantra is a way of life to achieve enlightenment and enjoy higher energy levels.

Tantra is a philosophy, a spiritual system, and an art form, as well as a way of life. It is related to Hinduism, Buddhism and the Chinese Tao. It is a doctrine very difficult to define, but by practicing it you become one with the universe and reach spiritual enlightenment. Tantra is to move the energy through, inside and outside the energy centers, align the energy with the couple, and therefore exchange energy between them, either having sex, hugging or just sit next to each other. In tantric sex, it is sought to conserve and concentrate the sexual energies to reach higher levels of energy.

To increase your levels of energy, practice conscious and intentional sacred sexuality.

8. <u>Hobbies</u>

Did you know that doing what you like is very effective to recharge your energy?

Hobbies are pleasurable activities to keep us entertained for a while. The energy that generates to make a pleasurable activity helps us to automatically recharge our energy.

To increase your levels of energy, discover and enjoy your hobbies.

9. <u>Love</u>

Did you know that love is an energy force?

Love is a decision, and a biochemical process that starts in the crust cerebral, passes to the neurons and from there to the endocrine system, giving rise to intense physiological responses. Dopamine and norepinephrine are segregated when we are in love. Actions related to being "in love" recharge our energy.

To increase your energy fall in love every day, have passion for life.

10. *Read*

Did you know that our body uses energy to read?

Did you know that what you read influences your energy levels?

Reading is the procedure by which people de-codify a message transmitted through the written code. The enormous value of the written expression lies in its endurance: the reader can reread a text as often as he wishes. The reading allows access to culture, tradition, information, knowledge of new cultures and critical thinking.

What we read is considered food for the mind, so we should be selective with the information that we receive. Reading is a vital activity in the educational process and therefore, the development of consciousness, the voluntary change of habits and the enjoyment of new lifestyles.

To increase your energy levels, read good books, search for positive topics that add value to your life.

11. *Listen*

Did you know that our body uses energy to listen?

Did you know that what you hear influences your levels of energy?

Did you know that listening stimulates your mind and affects your actions?

Listening positive sounds and information:

The ear is one of the first senses developed in a baby inside the womb and hence the importance of knowing how we are affected by what we hear.

Hearing negative things (as for example stories, songs with messages of anger or too much violence, sadness, fights, scolding) causes an energy waste, even if you don't notice it. On the other hand, through listening you can absorb the positive sounds, meaning messages and words related to the love, joy, harmony, etc., which increase your energy, recharging your brain, your body, and your mind.

Quiet time / Silent Retreat

A silent retreat/ quiet time is an opportunity for any person to set aside time to listen to the voice of God and hear what is in their own heart. Retreats can last a single day or up to thirty days, giving you a chance to unplug from the outside world and recharge your spiritual batteries.

To increase your energy levels, listen to constructive information and enjoy quiet time. Be selective.

12. *Associating with energetically conscious people*

Did you know that other people affect your energy frequency?

Did you know that there are energy vampires that just want to drain your energy?

Social intelligence is the ability to know how to relate. The concept of "social intelligence" was first used by psychologist Edward Thorndike in 1920, when he wrote an article highlighting the importance of interpersonal relationships.

It's important to partner with people with energy consciousness. You're the average of the five people you spend most of the time with. But, what does it mean?

If the 5 people are people who inspire the best of you, you will be growing and advancing in a constant way. But if your group of 5, they are not on the same frequency, it will be very difficult for you to achieve what you want.

Tell me who you walk with and your energy will say who you are...

To increase your energy levels, associate with energetically conscious people.

13. *Generate Passive Income*

Did you know that our body uses energy during the process of generating income?

Did you know that your relationship with money influences your energy levels?

Did you know that economic stress weakens your immune system?

The development of a system that generates passive income frees your time from the money equation, so you earn time to invest in activities that increase your levels of energy.

In addition, be able to satisfy your material needs and tastes produce energy, especially if the income is generated passively. Understanding the concept of passive income and how to develop it is vital in the energy process.

Robert Kiyosaki explains, in his book *Cashflow Quadrants*, that there are four ways to earn money: 1. Get money directly from being employed, 2. Work independently or own a small business and get money for services performed, 3. Owning a larger company with systems and getting money from your earnings, or 4. Invest in companies and get investment profit.

Passive or residual income generates profits no matter what you do during the day. Instead, active or linear income generates earnings in exchange for their work.

For information about Enagic, our passive income system, visit www.DRWinstitute.org

To increase your energy levels, integrate a system that generates passive income into your life or business.

14. *Living your Life Purpose*

Did you know that living your life purpose strengthens your immune system?

Did you know that living your life purpose influences your energy levels?

Discovering and living your life purpose is an energy generator. When you get up, you feel energized because you are doing what you know you were created to do.

Your life purpose is the statement that sustains your productivity, and the generation of energy. The life purpose is the combination of the passion (motivation), the potential (gifts and talents) and profit (economic engine). Only when a person achieves the intersection of the three will fulfill their destiny by living a life with a particular purpose and enjoying the results of creating energy consciousness, vitality, harmony, and alignment.

To increase your energy levels, discover and consciously live your life purpose.

15. *Living a holistic lifestyle*

Did you know that a holistic lifestyle positively influences your energy levels?

Did you know about the biological clock?

An option to live a holistic lifestyle is to align yourself to the biological clock described in Oriental medicine.

The practical utility of following the biological clock is energy efficiency and optimum performance of the human body and its systems.

- 3:00am – 5:00am: *Lungs Meridian*. Deep Sleep. Also recommended to make special breathing exercises accompanied by ***meditation and/or prayer***, to improve the oxygenation of the organism and to start the day with a clean and fresh mind.
- 5:00am – 7:00am: *Large Intestine Meridian*. Time to get up, drink a glass of ***water*** at room temperature and meet the natural needs of elimination.

- 7:00am – 9:00am: *Stomach Meridian*: Absorption of nutrients in the stomach. Ideal for having breakfast and nourishing the organism with an *energy diet.*

- 9:00am – 11:00am: *Spleen Meridian* is active; food is converted into blood and energy to nourish the muscles. The best hours to study, *work and build a passive income system*.

- 11.00am – 1:00pm: *Heart Meridian*, Lunchtime according to the *energy diet*, according to Chinese Traditional Medicine the heart also nourishes the mind and spirit, this is also a good time to revitalize the spirit, converse, and share.

- 1:00pm – 3:00pm: *Small Intestine Meridian*, the small intestine works by separating and distributing the digested nutrients. *Walk or physical activity* is advisable.

- 3:00pm – 5:00pm: *Bladder Meridian, **Work***. These are ideal hours for work or study. It Is advisable to drink tea to help the expulsion of toxins from the body and eating light foods at dinner.

- 5:00pm – 7:00pm: *Kidney Meridian*. Time for therapies, meditation, and introspection, discussing topics that have to do with philosophical and ethical principles, *Read and Listen* to Music.

- 7:00pm a 9:00pm: *Pericardium Meridian* in Chinese Medicine; this meridian drive loving activity and *sacred sexuality*, it also protects the heart by giving it inspiration, is a good time for interpersonal relationships to comfort the shared emotions with others and the collective spirit.

- 9:00pm – 11:00pm: *Triple Heater Meridian*, comprises the 3 main systems, oxygenation, circulation, digestion and energy assimilation. Unnecessary and toxic chemicals are eliminated through the organism's lymphatic system. A *meditation and/or prayer* in a quiet state is recommended.
- 11:00pm – 1:00am: *Gallbladder Meridian*. *Sleep* and Rest.
- 1:00am – 3:00am: *Liver Meridian*. The most important time for the rest of mind and metabolism, currently the energy of the liver cleanses the emotions the mind and the blood.

To increase your energy levels, it is advisable to consciously align yourself with the biological clock and live a holistic life.

Exercise:

1. What options are viable for you?

2. What options would you like to explore in detail?

3. Which options for increasing your energy can you integrate into your lifestyle immediately?

Part III

Energy Harmony

Unblock and Protect Your Energy

Objective:

The objective of this chapter is to facilitate *Energy Harmony* offering options for unblocking and protect your energy.

Unblock Your Energy

Lack of emotional intelligence causes emotions not to be handled in a healthy way and therefore result in energy stagnation. In accordance with Chinese Medicine, those stagnations are associated with diseases and physical health conditions. Identifying the emotions and exploring options to manage them in a healthier way is important to avoid and/or minimize energy stagnations.

1. Fear

Fear is an emotion characterized by an intense unpleasant feeling provoked by the perception of danger, real or supposed, present, future or even past.

Fear blocks the first energy center or chakra, located at on the perineum, between the genitals and the anus; affecting the power of survival and depleting your skeletal system.

Fear causes significant energy wasting affecting our health specifically at the central nervous system, adrenals glands, lymphatic system, male reproduction system, prostate, large intestine, coccyx, sacrum, bones, teeth, fingernails, legs, and arms. The energy blockage caused by fear can cause sciatica, constipation, ovarian problems, uterus, prostate problems, varicose veins, immune disorders, and the possibility of hemorrhoids.

To minimize or prevent energy blockages in the first energy center is vital to learn how to manage fear through the development of self-esteem and the gift of Fear of the Lord. Clearly establishing the level of risk that you are willing to assume before new experiences is a fundamental part of the process of energy harmonization. If after evaluating the risk associated with, you understand that it is not justified take the risk... It is ok!!!!

Learning to say "Yes" or "No" is a fundamental part of the energy harmonization process. There's a big difference between saying "Yes" or "No" out of fear and saying it with confidence.

2. Guilt

Guilt is an emotion associated with breaking rules (family, religious, natural, etc.) or by the thought of committing such acts.

Guilt blocks the second chakra, located at the base of the lumbar spine, midway between the navel and the pubic bone; affecting the power of creativity and depleting your reproductive system.

Guilt causes significant energy wear that affects our health specifically at the female reproductive organs, bladder, large intestine, pelvis, buttocks, and third lumbar to the sacrum. The energy blockage caused by guilt can cause lumbar tension, lumbar and pelvic pain, sciatica, kidney and bladder infections, immune system disorders, chronic fatigue, impotence, frigidity, irritable bowel, cancer, and diabetes.

To minimize or prevent energy blockages in the second energy center, it is vital to learn to handle guilt with forgiveness and the gift of mercy. Recognize that no one is perfect and that we all can improve is fundamental in the process of energy harmonization.

3. Shame

Shame is a conscious emotion of dishonor, misfortune or condemnation. Feeling ashamed is very common. Feelings of inferiority and lack of knowledge are the main causes of shame.

Shame blocks the third chakra that sits right above the navel, affecting the power of learning and depleting the digestive system.

Shame causes significant energy wear that affects our health specifically in the pancreas, liver, gallbladder, spleen, kidney, adrenal glands, stomach, small intestine, and the rib cage. The energy blockage caused by the shame can cause problems related to respiratory, immunologic, hormonal and digestive systems, ulcers, gallstones, heartburn, diabetes, hypoglycemia, tumors, anorexia, bulimia, hepatitis, cirrhosis, and arthritis.

To minimize or prevent energy blockages in the third energy center it is vital to learn how to manage shame through education and the gift of knowledge. Remember, our knowledge is limited, we do not know what we do not know, the important thing is to decide to learn and give us the opportunity of expanding our knowledge.

Recognize that we don't know everything and give us the opportunity to explore options is a fundamental part of energy harmony.

4. Sadness and Grief

Sadness or Grief is a normal and healthy response to a loss. There are many causes of loss, sadness, and pain in our lives. It is important to recognize that feeling sad is normal and is part of a grieving process. What is not normal is to live with sadness by blocking and wasting our energy.

When we talk about the grieving process, most of the time we refer to the 5 stages of the duel identified by

Elisabeth Kübler-Ross. Kübler-Ross was a psychiatrist who studied how people who had been diagnosed with a terminal illness grieved for health loss (Kübler-Ross, 1972). She identified the following 5 stages of the duel:

A. Denial:

"This is not happening. Not to me."

B. Anger:

"Why is it happening? Who is to blame?"

C. Bargaining:

"I Will Make a change in my life only if that means that this won't happen to me."

D. Depression:

"I don't care Anymore."

E. Acceptance:

"I am at peace with what is happening."

The sadness blocks the fourth chakra that lies right behind your heart, affecting the power of love and depleting the cardiovascular system.

The sadness causes an energy blockage affecting the heart, circulation, lungs, rib cage, thoracic spine, thymus, breasts, esophagus, arms, shoulders, and hands. The energy blockage caused by sadness can cause heart disease, asthma, lung disease, and breast problems, chest spinal problems, pneumonia, hypertension, stroke, angina pectoris, and arthritis.

To minimize or avoid energy blockages it is vital to learn to manage sadness and grief through gratefulness and the gift of fortitude. Building the strength to identify and handle our losses is fundamental in the development of energy harmony.

5. Distrust

Distrust is the emotion associated with not perceiving the truth, or we can tell the truth.

Distrust blocks the fifth chakra which is located at the back of the throat – affecting the power of communication and depleting the endocrine system.

The energy blockage caused by distrust can cause problems in the throat, voice, gums, teeth, thyroid disorders, flu, or colds, chronic infections and allergic reactions.

To minimize or prevent energy blockages in the fifth energy center it is vital to learn to manage mistrust through communication and the gift of the council. Being able to express ourselves in an open and honest way is a fundamental part of the development of energy harmony.

6. Disappointment

Disappointment is an emotion caused by our expectations and illusions. These expectations have been created based on our education, culture, traditions, past experiences and religious beliefs.

The disappointment blocks the sixth chakra which is located on the forehead; affecting the power of judgement and depleting the nervous system.

The disappointment causes energy blockage that affects the brain, pituitary, pineal glands, eyes, ears, nose; causing headache, confused thinking, brain tumors, strokes, blindness, deafness, seizures, learning problems, spine problems, panic, and depression.

To minimize or prevent blockages of energy in the sixth energy center it is vital to learn how to manage disappointment by means of empathy and the gift of understanding. Recognizing that we are all different, understanding diversity in our society, and understanding that nothing is absolute, everything is 50/50 is a fundamental part of the development of energy harmony.

7. Attachments

Attachments is an emotion that is defined as an intense affective bond that affects the sense of freedom and creates codependency. Codependency occurs when two people are united because of deficiencies and unmet needs in the emotional aspect, such as being afraid of loneliness or lack of self-confidence.

Attachment blocks the seventh chakra, which is in the crown of the head; affecting the power of believe and depleting the immune system.

The energy blockage caused by attachments can cause musculoskeletal problems, skin disorders, depression, chronic fatigue, hypersensitivity to light, sound and environmental stimulation.

To minimize or prevent energy blockages in the seventh energy center it is vital to learn to manage attachments by means of love in freedom and the gift of wisdom. Learn to love and be loved freely is vital to minimize the energy blockage caused by emotional attachments.

Valuing your energy arises as a result of knowing and experiencing the benefits of high energy. ***Don't let anything or anyone steal your energy***. You can consciously decide to invest energy but never waste your energy. Energy is too precious to waste.

Protect Your Energy

The model of *Holistic Emotional Intelligence* describes eight (8) health dimensions. Each dimension can be affected by emotional triggers. To protect our energy, we must identify the cause of the triggers, educate ourselves in the three options for consciously managing the triggers: illuminate, reduce dosage or eliminate.

1. Illuminate: Consciously invest energy in a person or situation to produce positive changes.
2. Reduce dosage: Consciously reduce the exposure time to the trigger given the case that cannot be eliminated.
3. Eliminate: Decide to avoid total exposure to the trigger.

Triggers may arise in any of the **Eight (8) Holistic Health Dimensions**:

1. Individual Health: "I Am"

Individual Health refers to "I am". Be aware of who you are and be able to be you is essential in holistic health. Living in a fake is an energy expense not justified.

The three aspects that integrate individual health are life purpose, fundamental values, and gifts/talents.

a. Life Purpose: Identifies the way forward during our existence and should be the combination of your passion, your talents, and your economic engine.

b. Core Values: The non-negotiable truth of a person and the guide in decision making.

c. Gifts and Talents: A series of natural skills given to you for the optimal performance of your life purpose.

The internal conflict caused by not having defined your individual health is an emotional trigger that causes energy stagnation and energetic wear.

It is recommended to meet with a qualified and certified Holistic Emotional Intelligence Coach© to explore options and design a plan of action to reduce energy leaks in the area of Individual Health.

2. Emotional Health: "I Feel"

Emotional Health refers to "I feel". Being aware of what we feel and being able to express it in a healthy way offers us an advantage in the handling of emotions.

Three aspects integrate emotional health: memories, attachments, and detonators. Lack of tools to handle these three aspects can cause a significant leak in our energy levels.

a. Emotional Memories: Events create memories that can be retrieved consciously or unconsciously. The positive memories serve us to recharge our energy, on the contrary, negative memories wear and block us. Avoid wasting your time and energy turning the negative memories into your head. Learn from them and let them go. Live thankful for the lived time and learning experience. Not handling the emotional memories in a healthy way causes energy stagnation and energetic wear.

b. Emotional Attachments: Attachments steal our freedom and make us slaves of unhealthy situations. Learn to love in freedom, and to respect the right of the freedom of every human being. Minimize the desire of controlling everything and everyone. Not handling healthy way causes energy stagnation and energetic wear.

c. Detonators: The emotional detonators are stimuli that generate unconscious answers consuming our energy. Don't handle the emotional detonators in a healthy way causes energy stagnation and energetic wear.

It is recommended to meet with a qualified and certified Holistic Emotional Intelligence Coach© to explore options and design an action plan to reduce energy expenditure in the area of emotional health.

3. Intellectual Health: "I Know"

Intellectual health can be defined as what I know or the ability to learn. The style of learning of an individual indicates how he or she recovers and retains the information better. The VAK Learning model of Bandler and Grinder It comprises three methods of sensory Learning: visual (vison), auditory (sound) and kinesthetic (touch or movement).

a. Visual: People who prefer to learn visually can be classified into two groups: linguistic or spatial. People who prefer to learn in this way tend to associate new information with mental images.

b. Auditory: These individuals like to receive new information and instructions through listening and speaking. People with this learning preference can enjoy activities involving exchanges of ideas, debates and other vocal exchanges that take place among people.

c. Kinesthetic: Kinesthetic individuals can be classified as touch or movement dependent. These people perform better when they are encouraged to be active.

Identifies which areas of your life you want to develop, and/or which areas you want to master. Not recognizing our continuous learning ability causes energy stagnation and energetic wear.

It is recommended to meet with a qualified and certified Holistic Emotional Intelligence Coach© to explore options and design a plan to minimize energy expenditure in the area of intellectual health.

4. Mental Health: "I Understand"

Mental health is basically the combination of the individual, emotional and intellectual health. It's relative to "Who am I", "How I feel", and "What do I understand"; affecting our response to crises and situations in life.

Mental health has three components in the holistic model: consciousness, clarity, and stability.

a. Consciousness is an aptitude or ability to discern that manifests itself in a conscious state.

b. Mental Clarity is the ability to think clearly and facilitates the making of personal and professional decisions.

c. Mental Stability is the ability to handle your emotions and plan your response, resist the impulses and operate in a flexible and at the same time-controlled way.

Not maintaining stable mental health causes energy stagnation and energetic wear.

It is recommended to meet with a qualified and certified Holistic Emotional Intelligence Coach© to explore options and design a plan to minimize energy expenditure in the mental health area.

5. Health Physical: "I Act"

Physical health is the result of how your body works. The human body is a complex mechanism of precision, whose performance and performance depend on the optimal performance and harmonic coordination of the organs and systems that compose it. Therefore, to know as emotions affect the body is fundamental in the development of energy harmony.

The human body has eleven (11) anatomical systems/apparatus: digestive, endocrine, respiratory, integumentary, nervous, urinary, muscular, skeletal (bone), immune, cardiovascular and reproductive.

1. *Digestive System "The Sense of Taste"*

Digestion is a physiological process that includes ingesting food, assimilating nutrients, and eliminating waste. Digestion can help to increase or reduce energy. The sense of taste is very complex. By means of the sense of taste, we receive a stimulus that are translated into information.

What you eat create and recover emotional memories; what you eat it is detonated by emotion, and how you eat is influenced by emotions.

The eating can increase or reduce our energy.

The lack of knowledge and abuse of the digestive system cause energy stagnation and energetic wear.

It is recommended to meet with a qualified and certified Holistic Emotional Intelligence Coach© to

explore options and design a plan to minimize the energy expenditure caused by the digestive system.

2. *Respiratory System "The Sense of smell"*

The respiratory system is fundamental in our energy, it can help to increase or reduce energy. The sense of smell is very sensitive. Through the sense of smell, we receive stimulus that translate into information.

What we smell creates or recovers emotional memories, the way we breathe is influenced by our emotions.

The breathing can increase or reduce our energy.

The lack of knowledge and abuse of the respiratory system cause energy stagnation and energetic wear.

It is recommended to meet with a qualified and certified Holistic Emotional Intelligence Coach© to explore options and design a plan to minimize the energy expenditure caused by the respiratory system.

3. *Integumentary System "The Sense of touch"*

Touch is one of our basic senses. The skin is the largest organ in our body and receives a lot of information and stimuli.

What we touch create and recover emotional memories, and how we touch is influenced by our emotions.

The touching can increase or reduce the energy.

The lack of knowledge and abuse of the integumentary system cause energy stagnation and energetic wear.

It is recommended to meet with a qualified and certified Holistic Emotional Intelligence Coach to explore options and design a plan to minimize the energy expenditure caused by the integumentary system.

4. *Nervous System "The Sense of Information"*

The nervous system is a structure to receive, interpret and respond to information. The information received sends stimulus that detonate our emotional responses.

What we see and we hear creates and recovers emotional memories, as we look, and we hear is influenced by emotions.

The nervous responses can increase or reduce energy.

The lack of knowledge and abuse of the nervous system cause energy stagnation and energetic wear.

It is recommended to meet with a qualified and certified Holistic Emotional Intelligence Coach© to explore options and design a plan to minimize the energy expenditure caused by the nervous system.

5. *Endocrine system: "The sense of communication"*

The endocrine system produces hormones that are released into the blood and that regulate some of the functions of the body including mood, growth, and metabolism.

Hormones are released by the influence of emotional events and memories, and hormones influence the manifestation of emotions.

The hormones can increase or reduce energy.

The lack of knowledge and abuse of the endocrine system cause energy stagnation and energetic wear.

It is recommended to meet with a qualified and certified Holistic Emotional Intelligence Coach© to explore options and design a plan to minimize the energy expenditure caused by the endocrine system.

6. *Immune System: "The Sense of defense"*

The immune system protects against diseases identifying and eliminating pathogenic and cancerous cells.

Immunity is influenced by emotional events and memories; immunity influences the manifestation of emotions.

The immunity can increase or reduce energy.

The lack of knowledge and abuse of the immune system cause energy stagnation and energetic wear.

It is recommended to meet with a qualified and certified Holistic Emotional Intelligence Coach© to explore options and design a plan to minimize the energy expenditure caused by the immune system.

7. *Muscular System: "The sense of movement"*

The muscular system muscular allows the skeleton to move, to remain stable and to shape the body. The muscular system serves as a protection for the proper functioning of the digestive system and other vital organs. The human body is composed of about 600 muscles. The muscles transform the chemical energy into the ability to carry out work.

The movement is influenced by events and emotional memories, movement increases the manifestation of emotions.

The movement can increase or reduce energy.

The lack of knowledge and abuse of the muscular system cause energy stagnation and energetic wear.

It is recommended to meet with a qualified and certified Holistic Emotional Intelligence Coach© to explore options and design a plan to minimize the energy expenditure caused by the muscular system.

8.   *Skeletal System: "The Sense of structural support"*

The skeletal system serves as a structural support and protection of internal organs. The human body consists of about 206 bones: crane 22, spine 26; upper extremities and chests 64; and lower limbs and hips 62.

The posture is influenced by events and emotional memories, the posture increases the manifestation of emotions.

The posture can increase or reduce energy.

The lack of knowledge and abuse of the skeletal system cause energy stagnation and energetic wear.

It is recommended to meet with a qualified and certified Holistic Emotional Intelligence Coach© to explore options and design a plan to minimize the energy expenditure caused by the skeletal system.

9. *Reproductive System: "The Sense of creation"*

The reproductive system is related to sexual reproduction. It's a vital part of our energy consciousness and the enjoyment of Mobius or energy alignment.

Sexuality is influenced by events and emotional memories, and sexuality influences the manifestation of emotions.

Sexuality can increase or reduce energy.

The lack of knowledge and abuse of the reproductive system cause energy stagnation and energetic wear.

It is recommended to meet with a qualified and certified Holistic Emotional Intelligence Coach© to explore options and design a plan to minimize the energy expenditure caused by the reproductive system.

10. *Urinary System: "The Sense of elimination"*

The urinary system has the function of expelling the waste that has left the digestive process.

The urgency and frequency of urination are influenced by emotional events and memories; and the urgency and frequency of urinating influences the manifestation of emotions.

The urgency and frequency of urination can increase or reduce energy.

The lack of knowledge and abuse of the urinary system cause energy stagnation and energetic wear.

It is recommended to meet with a qualified and certified Holistic Emotional Intelligence Coach© to explore options and design a plan to minimize the energy expenditure caused by the urinary system.

11. *Circulatory System: "The Sense of transportation"*

The circulatory system is a closed group of venous and arterial connections that transport blood to the organs of the body.

The heartbeat is influenced by emotional events and memories; the heartbeat influences the manifestation of emotions.

The heartbeat can increase or reduce energy.

The lack of knowledge and abuse of the circulatory system cause energy stagnation and energetic wear.

It is recommended to meet with a qualified and certified Holistic Emotional Intelligence Coach© to explore options and design a plan to minimize the energy expenditure caused by the circulatory system.

In summary, emotions poorly managed cause diseases. In recent years, several studies have confirmed that our emotions are linked to our physical state. Our body always emits a reaction in accordance with what we think, feel and do. This is how the mind-body connection is given.

The following guide aims to help you to detect what kind of emotion may be causing your pain or chronic illness to look for viable and effective options to fix the problem.

1. Muscle Aches: These kinds of pains refer to our ability to flow with our daily situations.
2. Headaches: Headaches relate with important decision makings in the life.
3. Neck Aches: This type of pain is related to forgiveness... If you have a lot of pain in your neck or areas close to it, sit back and think about what you need to forgive.

4. Gum Aches: If we talk about emotions that cause disease, insecurity and lack of commitment are associated with pain in the gums.

5. Shoulder Pain: The pain in the shoulders is associated with the excess of emotional burden upon us.

6. Stomach Aches: If you suffer chronically from stomach aches without having clear nutritional reasons to suffer from them, you may be needing to seriously question what it is that you cannot digest at all well in your life or what is too hard to accept.

7. Upper Back Pain: Chronic pain at the top of your back speaks to us about how little we are supported or loved we feel.

8. Pain in the sacrum and coccyx: The pains in these parts of the body are often emotionally associated with situations that tense and worry us.

9. Pain in the Elbows: Pain in the elbows is often associated with resistance to change.

10. Pain in the arms in general: Is clear evidence that there is a huge burden in your life that is not letting you move forward; it can be a person or a situation.

11. Pain in the Hands: Hands are our means of contact with what surrounds us; commonly the pain of the hands is often associated with

something that wants but for some reason it's getting very difficult to reach. The pain of hands can be also associated with the difficulty of letting loose something very dear to you.

12. Pain in the hips: The difficulty of adapting to the changes are usually associated directly with the pain of the hips.

13. Muscle and Joint Pain: Often associated with a lack of mobility and experience; to the fear of new adventures and challenges.

14. Knee Pain: The pain in the knees usually is associated with the over-demand with oneself.

15. Pain in the Teeth: The pain in the teeth arises when we don't feel comfortable in a situation and we don't find a way to deal with it.

16. Ankle Pain: Usually, ankle pain is usually associated with a lack of pleasure in your life.

17. Foot Pain: Foot pain is associated with depression and low mood. Feet are very sensitive body points, capable of to immediately detect this kind of negative emotion in us.

The lack of knowledge and abuse of our physical body cause energy stagnation and energetic wear.

It is recommended to meet with a qualified and certified Holistic Emotional Intelligence Coach© to explore options and design an action plan to reduce energy expenditure in the area of physical health.

6. *Social Health "I Interact"*

Social health is defined by the interaction with other people at varying levels of influence in our lives. Every human being vibrates at a different energy frequency since it has been exposed to various experiences and situations.

a. Family: Love "Strict" Family love. Humans united by blood bonds.

b. Friends: Love "philia" The Brotherly love. In the Book _Resolved_, _13 resolutions for the life_, Orrin Woodward shares with us eight principles for a true friendship.

1. The true friendships are formed around the same interests, points of view or tastes, enjoying the common bonds that unite them.

2. True friends are accepted as they are, loving themselves regardless of their imperfections.

3. True friends accept each other, protect each other's weaknesses, and applaud their virtues.

4. True friends appreciate each other, motivate themselves, help each other, and believe in each other's talents and abilities.

5. True friends listen with empathy, learn from the hopes, dreams, fears, and difficulties of the other.

6. True friends celebrate successes of the other and feel proud of the other's accomplishments without the minimum hint of envy.

7. True friends are trustworthy, keep the shared secrets with impeccable honor and respect and understand that the gossip separates best friends.

8. True friends are loyal, respect and defend the character, the reputation on and the motives of the other if the truth allows, and they face any concern or problem between them so that the misunderstandings no increase.

c. Couple: Love "Eros" Sensual love. A couple relationship should be based in the eight principles of true friendship, plus emotional, physical and energetic intimacy. Trust, respect and admiration are a must in a couple relationship. To achieve emotional intimacy, we must integrate the pillars of Holistic Emotional Intelligence in our relationship, and to achieve a physical intimacy we must value and respect our body and our partner's. To achieve energetic intimacy with our partner we must develop vitality and harmony at the individual level. The book "*Sexual Intelligence*", offers education in the subject of sexuality.

d. Work: Relationships at work are an energy challenge. Either coworkers or customers may be vibrating at a different energy frequency from ours or with less wavelength causing wear energy. It is vital to remember the strategy of social consciousness: *illuminate, eliminate or reduce the dosage.*

    i. We can become a change agent positively impacting the lives of our co-workers and clients;

    ii. We can explore options to change jobs or department by eliminating the exposure(n) to such frequencies, or

> iii. we can explore options to reduce contact with those toxic people.

The conscious practice of Holistic Emotional Intelligence Holistic provides us the strength to make changes in our life that minimize the energy drainage caused by people vibrating at lower frequency.

e. Community: The level of participation in our community activities is a personal decision. Therefore, it must be a conscious decision based on the energy impact that's going to cause in us. The community work can reload, drain or both. If we recharge, we are enjoying it and we have learned to handle the inherent triggers of interpersonal relationships. If it drains us, we must consciously evaluate the energy return of investment and take the decision on to reduce the dose or eliminate. If we recharge and drains us at once, we must evaluate the net of activity, and learn how to reduce the dosage, eliminate, or improve our techniques for the handling of detonators.

f. Environment: Our relationship with the environment should be symbiotic, or both sides getting benefits. Nature offers us natural resources for production of energy. We in return must protect the natural resources and Mother Earth in a conscious way. Flora and fauna are both a source of emotional and physical energy, is our duty to care for and protect resources.

Toxic relationships cause energy stagnation and energetic wear.

It is recommended to meet with a qualified and certified Holistic Emotional Intelligence Coach© to explore options and design an action plan to reduce energy expenditure in the area of social health.

7. *Financial Health "I Exchange"*

In holistic health we define financial health as the peace we feel in our relationship with money and finances. Orrin Woodward's book *Resolved, 13 Resolutions for Life*, presents ten principles that can help people gain knowledge in finance and reduce energy waste caused by financial stress.

1. Identify net income/revenue
2. Documents all expenses
3. Set a financial goal
4. Never finance anything that depreciates
5. Set a price limit on spontaneous purchases
6. Pay off credit card debt and use cash whenever is possible

7. Wipe out all consumer debt before starting to save
8. Know the difference between an investment and an expense
9. Focus on quality of life and peace of mind
10. Be a blessing to others

Time is the only limited resource and to use it to generate income enslaves us. The author Orrin Woodward shares with us that building a business asset is the solution and explains that the fastest way to achieve this is to leverage the left quadrants of the cash flow for short-term security and those on the right to achieve long-term goals.

The lack of Financial Literacy cause energy stagnation and energetic wear.

It is recommended to meet with a qualified and certified Holistic Emotional Intelligence Coach© to explore options and design an action plan to reduce energy expenditure in the area of financial health.

8. *Spiritual Health "I Believe"*

Every human being is responsible for their beliefs and to practice their spirituality. Human diversity allows us to accept ourselves with our differences of thought and belief. The important factor is that you do not have internal conflicts that wear your energy. Universal Energy, Chi, Qi, Human Essence or Holy Spirit, as you prefer to call it is the vital force that keep us alive.

The lack of spirituality cause energy stagnation and energetic wear.

It is recommended to meet with a qualified and certified Holistic Emotional Intelligence Coach© to explore options and design an action plan to reduce energy expenditure in the area of spiritual health.

Each area of holistic health may present triggers that cause energy leaks and blockages. Valuing our energy and its benefits helps us to identify areas of improvement and fix it.

Exercise:

Identify areas of Stagnation Energy:
Evaluate each area using the following key:
1 = Not acceptable
2 = Small
3 = ok
4 = well
5 = Wonderful
6 = Excellent

Area	1	2	3	4	5	6
Individual Health						
Life Purpose						
Core Values						
Gifts and Talents						
Emotional Health						
Emotional Triggers						
Emotional Memories						
Emotional Attachments						
Intellectual Health						
Formal Education						
Informal Education						
Mental Health						
Clarity						
Stability						
Awareness						

Area	1	2	3	4	5	6
Physical Health						
Digestive System						
Respiratory System						
Integumentary System						
Nervous System						
Endocrine System						
Immune System						
Muscular System						
Skeletal System						
Reproductive System						
Urinary System						
Circulatory System						
Social Health						
Intimacy						
Family						
Friends						
Work						
Community						
Environment						
Financial Health						
Income						
Expenses						
Net Difference						
Emergency Fund						
Debts						
Savings						

Inversions						
Retirement Plan						
Spiritual Health						
Peace						
Practices						

Identifies the emotions associated with each area:

7= Attachments

6 = Disappointment

5 = Distrust

4 = Sadness and grief

3 = Shame

2 = Fault

1 = Fear

Area	1	2	3	4	5	6	7
Individual Health							
Emotional Health							
Intellectual Health							
Mental Health							
Physical Health							
Social Health							
Financial Health							
Spiritual Health							

Part IV

Energy Alignment

Expand and Enjoy Energy

Objective:

The objective of this chapter is to facilitate *Energy Alignment* offering options to expand and enjoy your energy.

Enjoy and Expand Your Energy

Enjoyment of functional and healthy interpersonal relationships that are mutually satisfactorily is a conscious task based on energy. The energy alignment that is enjoyed by being in the presence of a human being that has developed energy awareness and practice the Holistic Emotional Intelligence techniques is indescribable. Whether on a personal or professional level, the goal is to enjoy the energy alignments and achieve higher levels of energy.

At the professional level, whether customers or coworkers, being in positive environments increases productivity. In this case, we can be more selective with our environment and interpersonal relationships.

On the personal level, it would be ideal to enjoy a positive environment where every member of our family has developed energy consciousnesseses. We know that many times it is not the case, each member of our family is on a different energy journey. It is important to recognize when it is necessary to recharge our energy. Many times, we must be in the presence of our family by dose or have limited meetings to not exhaust our energy levels, while we give them time to develop energy awareness.

In the personal level, our friends, a true friendship is not an energetic wear. A true friendship that meets the following eight principles becomes one of the most effective ways to enjoy energetic alignment.

- True friends form around shared insights
- True friends accept one another
- True friends approve of one another
- True friends appreciate one another
- True friends celebrate one another's success
- True friends listen with empathy
- True friends are trustworthy
- True friends are loyal

The best way to find an energy friend is to be one of them. This is accomplished by developing the art and science of friendship, and of course energy consciousness, vitality and harmony.

On a personal level, a relationship of intimacy should be a relationship based on energy alignment. A relationship where both parties have developed energy consciousness, vitality and harmony; and are committed to achieving higher energy levels in each encounter, despite their imperfect humanity. A relationship based on mutual respect, trust and admiration, where those are not negotiable.

Finally, alignment with the universal life energy is the main goal, the highest level of energy possible. There are close to 50 cultures around the world that have been identified the concept of life energy in one form or another; e.g., Ki (Japanese), Chi (Chinese), Prana (Sanskrit), Neyatoneyah (Lakota Sioux), Num (Kalahari Kung), Ruach or Roohah (Hebrew), Rooh (Persian), Lung (Tibetan), Holy Spirit (Christians) and so forth. The universal energy is pure and constant; therefore, it is the best energy source.

Although we can feel separated from everyone and everything because our energy vibrates at a different frequency from everything that exists, we can align ourselves with everything and everyone. Our energy connects, absorbs, interconnects and communicates with others here on Earth, as well as the incoming energies of the outer universe. Our job is to increase energy and keep it in harmony with the goal of enjoying energy alignment.

It is recommended to work with a certified coach in the Holistic Emotional Intelligence Coaching Method © to explore options and design a plan to enjoy energy alignment in your interpersonal relationships.

Exercise:

1. Are you enjoying energy alignment in any of the relationships?

2. Are your relationships functional?

3. Are your relationships healthy?

4. Are your relationships mutually satisfactory?

Part V

Energy Communion

Vibrate Higher and Experience Mobius

Objective:

The objective of this chapter is to facilitate Energetic Communion by offering options to vibrate higher and experience *Mobius.*

Vibrate higher and Experience *Mobius*

Mobius is an intimate experience of conscious, intentional, voluntary and mutual energy exchange; with the purpose of becoming one energy. It is a transitory moment that becomes eternal, where the body vibrates at high frequencies and perceives a separation from the tangible body. The separation of the energies is almost impossible after living this experience. It is like try to separate salt from sugar.

When we said conscious, we mean to be completely present without space to regret.

When we are intentional, we refer to knowing the purpose of exchanging our energy and essence.

When we are voluntary, we refer to free and spontaneous, in no way feel pressured or coerced. When we are mutual, we mean that both parties are in the same line and willing to give themselves in the same way.

To experience *Mobius,* you can choose two paths: individual or dual. The individual path refers to living the experience alone and offers you options for energetic communion with the source of universal energy. The dual path refers to living the experience accompanied and offers you options for energetic communion with other human beings. In order to achieve this level of energy you must develop energy consciousness, vitality, harmony and alignment. This will be a higher level, and energy doesn't lie.

Personally, living *Mobius* is a sacred experience, and a constant goal. Walking consciously in the energy world will give you the opportunity to live *Mobius* to the fullest. It's worth it! I assure!

Let's vibrate higher… it's all about energy – Dr. W

There are different philosophies and modalities to experience Mobius, as Theology of the Body and Tantra. It's important to evaluate and select the best option for you according to your values and beliefs.

It is recommended to work with a certified "coach" in the *Holistic Emotional Intelligence Coaching Method* © to explore options and design a plan to enjoy Energy Communion *Mobius*.

Conclusion

The intentional and conscious practice of *Holistic Emotional Intelligence* gives you tangible positive results such as; better health, more productivity and the enjoyment of mutually satisfactory interpersonal relationships.

The process of discovering and feeling your energy offers the **Energy Consciousness** needed to educate yourself and make changes in your lifestyle.

The process of increasing and recharging your energy offers the **Energy Vitality** needed to live to the fullest.

The process of unblocking and protecting your energy offers the **Energy Harmony** needed to handle emotional triggers in the eight dimensions of health.

The process of expanding and enjoying your energy offers the **Energy Alignment** needed to achieve exponential levels and enjoy mutually satisfying interpersonal relationships.

The process of raising your energy and experiencing Mobius offers the **Energy Communion** needed to vibrate at higher energy frequencies.

Learning and practicing *Holistic Emotional Intelligence* will allow you to vibrate higher and enjoy all the life experiences and adventures with an energetic perspective. In summary, you will be happier and enjoy PEACE!

Enjoy your journey in the world of energy. Keep discovering, experiencing, researching, learning and practicing techniques and modalities that allow you to vibrate higher; and remember,

What you do you want? What's your goal?

Set Your Mind… It's All About Energy and Energy Doesn't Lie!!! – Dr. W

BONUS

Holistic Emotional Intelligence Coaching Method ©

Holistic Emotional Intelligence Coaching Method©

The Holistic Emotional Intelligence Coaching Method© is a systematic communication model that allows us to be more effective in handling situations and emotional triggers. It's an encounter between a qualified and certified "coach" and the "client" with the purpose of working more efficiently on customer goals to reduce the energy stagnation and achieve higher levels of energy.

Holistic Emotional Intelligence Coaching Method© has four fundamental objectives:

1. Define clear Goals
2. Explore viable Options
3. Design strategic Plans
4. Offer Follow-Up

The scope of practice of the "coach" is to ask powerful questions and provide a safe and confidential space where the customer can express themselves, reflect, reconsider and objectively evaluate their own responses.

The client's role is, to be honest, and fully committed to the process.

The *Holistic Emotional Intelligence Coaching Method©* was developed and copyrighted by Dr. Wanda Bonet-Gascot. It is a sequence of seven steps to minimize energy consumption in conflict resolution, emotional trigger handling, and problem solving in any of the eight areas of holistic health.

Step # 1: Responsibility

Responsibility is the step to establish "who" oversees "what" in the coaching process.

The coach sets his/her responsibility in the meeting in a clear way and asks the customer what is the reason for the visit.

The client, on the other hand, express the reason of the meeting.

Step # 2: Honesty

Honesty is the step to clearly define goals and objectives.

The client should describe your current situation and your desired situation. In coaching terms, the point A and point B.

The coach facilitates the process to the client by means of powerful questions and active listening.

Step # 3: Commitment

Commitment is a step to establish the client's level of commitment in reaching the goals.

The coach should facilitate the establishment of the client's commitment level with its goal. Commitment is not with the coach, the commitment is with themselves, with achieving their goal.

The client must be 100% committed with his/her goals.

Step # 4: Creativity

Creativity is the skill to see opportunities, options, and solutions.

The coach should explore the client's creativity. Facilitate the process of exploring the options that the customer knows and does not remember or the options that the client doesn't know. The goal is to listen to our client in every sense of the word. Listen to the words, gestures, the tone of voice, body language, silences, and pauses.

Step # 5: Confidentiality

Confidentiality is the ability to share information and emotions in a healthy and safe way. This skill allows us to listen and express ourselves to a superior level listening during the process we call communication.

The coach will offer new options to the client.

The client must accept the offer of the coach. Remember the process of coaching the free and voluntary, the customer must express their availability to receive options and know that it is free to decide whether they are viable based on their reality.

Step # 6: Tolerance

Tolerance is associated with the level of risk that the person is willing to take. The person must invest time, effort and/or money.

Not all options are viable for all people, so it is a vital part of the coaching process that the customer chooses which options to be part of your plan of action. We know that for the plan to have results the person needs a strong reason, willpower and an instrument.

It's time to design the plan.

Step 7: Integrity and Initiative

It's time for action. And action begins from the moment when we make the decision to execute the plan. Action is a verb. Action is consistent and intentional. Action consists of a strategic.

Just thinking about how to improve doesn't change anything if a plan is not designed and action is taken.

For information about the *Holistic Emotional Intelligence©* Coach certification visit www. DRWinstitute.org

Additional Services:

Coaching: Individual / Group coaching session facilitated by a qualified and certified *Holistic Emotional Intelligence Coach©* in a safe and confidential environment.

Workshops: Class based on the concepts presented in this book.

Retreat: *All inclusive Energy Weekend Retreat,* transformational experience based on the *Holistic Emotional Intelligence©* model with the objective of facilitating energy consciousness, vitality, harmony, alignment and communion.

Holistic Emotional Intelligence Coach© Certification: Complete education that qualifies, certifies and empowers graduates to use the Holistic *Emotional Intelligence©* model.

Licensing Opportunity: Agreement that authorizes a *Holistic Emotional Intelligence Coach©* to share the *Holistic Emotional Intelligence©* model and profit from it.

For more information www.DRWinstitute.org

About the Author

Dr. Wanda Bonet-Gascot is the founder and director of operations at *DRW Life Skills Institute & Coaching School*, education center for personal and professional development at the Business Incubator of the University of Central Florida in Kissimmee, FL.

Her extensive education includes: Bachelor of Chemistry, Master of Business Administration, Master of Tantric Sexuality and a Doctorate in Holistic Nutrition. She is a licensed massage therapist specialized in energy modalities.

She collaborates with the University of Central Florida School of Medicine educating medical students in communication skills and emotional intelligence since 2009.

She is the author of the books "*Why am I not happy?*" (2012), "*Sexual Intelligence*" (2016) and the *Holistic Emotional Intelligence Model* (2013). She is a passionate energy practitioner, curious researcher and forever student. She loves traveling, and photography.

Dr. Bonet-Gascot is recognized for her commitment of sharing the Holistic Emotional Intelligence message in Central Florida and has received numerous awards for her work within the community.

References & Resources

Bonet-Gascot, W (2012) *Why am I not Happy?* Indiana: Palibrio.

Bonet-Gascot, W (2016) *Inteligencia Sexual*, Indiana: Palibrio.

Like breathing deeply. Retrieved 02-15-2018 from https://es.wikihow.com/respirar-profundamente

Body Aches are linked to emotional states. Retrieved 03-21-2019

http://www.viveconsalud.org/2017/06/24/19-dolores -en-el-cuerpo-que-estan-ligados-a-estados-emocionales/

Even, D (2008) *Energetic Medicine, Manual to achieve the energetic balance of the body for excellent health, joy, and vitality*. New York: Penguin Group.

The Heart This In the brain. Recovered 02-14-2018 Of https://bioemotionssite.wordpress.com/2017/11/03/ el-corazon-esta-en-el-cerebro/

The Dream Cycle. Retrieved 02-15-2018 from http://www.mejordormir.com/como_despertar_sin_sueno

Energetic Naps. Retrieved 02-15-2018 from Https://es.wikihow.com/tomar-siestas-energéticas

Health Benefits of fasting. Retrieved 04-03-2019 from https://www.globalhealingcenter.com/natural-health/health-benefits-of-fasting/

Importance of Reading. Retrieved 02-16-2018 from http://importancia.de/lectura/#ixzz57IWTDV2g

Woodward, O. (2013). *Financial Solvency*. North Carolina: Obstacles Press.

Woodward, (2015). *The Financial Matrix*. North Carolina: Obstacles Press.

Woodward, O. (2012) *Resolved*. North Carolina: Obstacles Press